The Inspired Mediterranean Meals Recipes

Super Simple Everyday Delicious Recipes To Boost Your Brain

Alison Russell

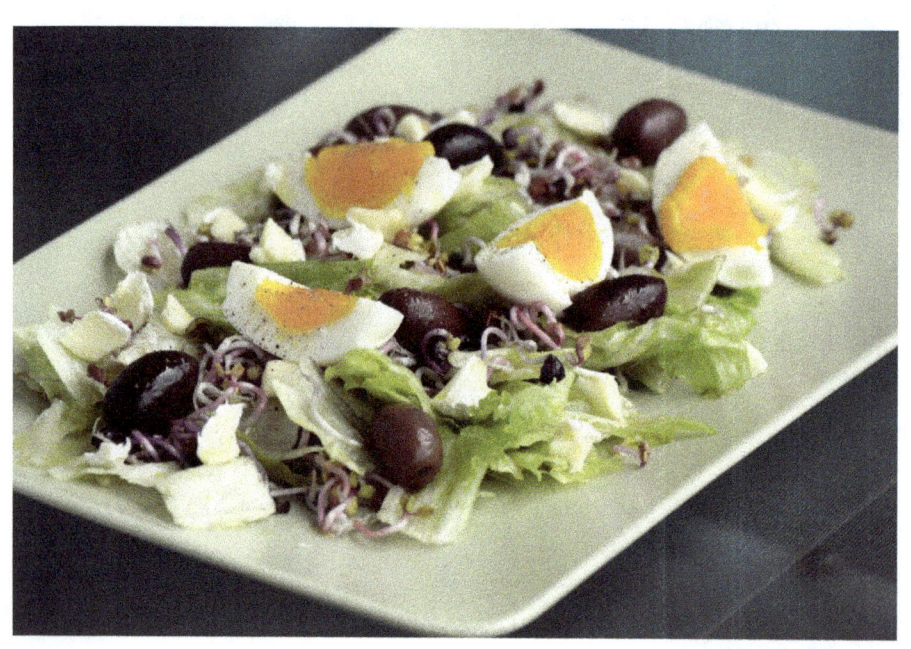

© **Copyright 2020 - All rights reserved.**

The content contained within this book may not be reproduced, duplicated or transmitted without direct written permission from the author or the publisher.

Under no circumstances will any blame or legal responsibility be held against the publisher, or author, for any damages, reparation, or monetary loss due to the information contained within this book. Either directly or indirectly.

Legal Notice:

This book is copyright protected. This book is only for personal use. You cannot amend, distribute, sell, use, quote or paraphrase any part, or the content within this book, without the consent of the author or publisher.

Disclaimer Notice:

Please note the information contained within this document is for educational and entertainment purposes only. All effort has been executed to present accurate, up to date, and reliable, complete information. No warranties of any kind are declared or implied. Readers acknowledge that the author is not engaging in the rendering of legal, financial, medical or professional advice. The content within this book has been derived from various sources. Please consult a licensed professional before attempting any techniques outlined in this book.

By reading this document, the reader agrees that under no circumstances is the author responsible for any losses, direct or indirect, which are incurred as a result of the use of information contained within this document, including, but not limited to, — errors, omissions, or inaccuracies.

Table of contents

Breakfast 9
    Avocado Smoothie 9
    Savory Breakfast Oatmeal 11
    Feta and Olive Scrambled Eggs 13
    Feta and Spinach Frittata 15
    Avocado and Egg Toast 17
    Tomato and Egg Breakfast Pizza 19
    Classic Shakshuka 21
    Parmesan Oatmeal with Greens 23
    Mediterranean Omelet 26
    Berry and Nut Parfait 28

Sides, Salads, and Soups 29
    Pumpkin Soup with Crispy Sage Leaves 29
    Mushroom Barley Soup 32
    Paella Soup 34
    Parmesan Roasted Red Potatoes 36
    Garlic Wilted Greens 39
    Sautéed Kale with Olives 40
    Balsamic Brussels Sprouts and Delicata Squash ... 42
    Green Beans with Tahini-Lemon Sauce 44

    Mixed Salad With Balsamic Honey Dressing 46

    Arugula and Fig Salad 48

Sandwiches, Pizzas, and Wraps 50

    Mediterranean Greek Salad Wraps 50

    Salmon Salad Wraps 52

    Baked Parmesan Chicken Wraps 54

    Eggplant, Spinach, and Feta Sandwiches 57

    Grilled Caesar Salad Sandwiches 59

    Green Veggie Sandwiches 61

    Pizza Pockets 63

    Mushroom-Pesto Baked Pizza 64

    Tuna and Hummus Wraps 66

    Chickpea Lettuce Wraps 68

Beans, Grains, and Pastas 70

    Minestrone Chickpeas and Macaroni Casserole 70

    Garlic and Parsley Chickpeas 72

    Black-Eyed Peas Salad with Walnuts 74

    Mashed Beans with Cumin 77

    Turkish Canned Pinto Bean Salad 79

    Fava and Garbanzo Bean Ful 81

    Triple-Green Pasta with Cheese 82

Caprese Pasta with Roasted Asparagus 84

Garlic Shrimp Fettuccine 86

Pesto Pasta 88

Poultry and Meats 90

Lamb Kofta (Spiced Meatballs) 90

Fish and Seafood 92

Baked Salmon with Tarragon Mustard Sauce 92

Baked Lemon Salmon 94

Glazed Broiled Salmon 95

Baked Salmon with Basil and Tomato 96

Honey-Mustard Roasted Salmon 97

Baked Fish with Pistachio Crust 98

Sole Piccata with Capers 100

Haddock with Cucumber Sauce 102

Crispy Herb Crusted Halibut 104

Breakfast

Avocado Smoothie

Prep time: 2 minutes | Cook time: 0 minutes | Serves 2

1 large avocado

1½ cups unsweetened coconut milk

2 tablespoons honey

1. Place all ingredients in a blender and blend until smooth and creamy.
2. Serve immediately.

Per Serving

calories: 686 | fat: 57.6g | protein: 6.2g | carbs: 35.8g | fiber: 10.7g | sodium: 35mg

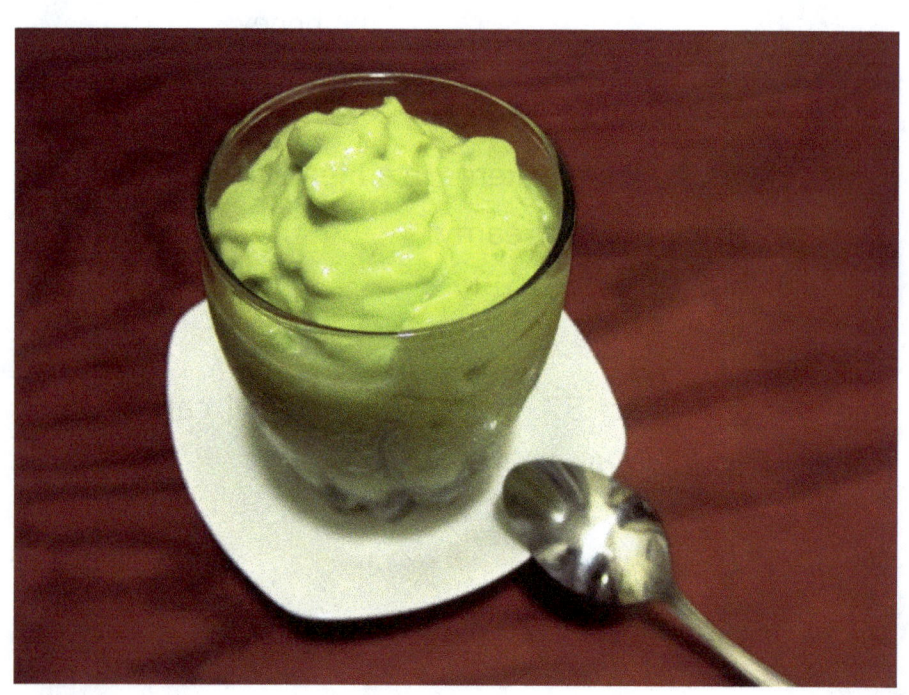

Savory Breakfast Oatmeal

Prep time: 5 minutes | Cook time: 15 minutes | Serves 2

½ cup steel-cut oats

1 cup water

1 medium cucumber, chopped

1 large tomato, chopped

1 tablespoon olive oil

Pinch freshly grated Parmesan cheese

Sea salt and freshly ground pepper, to taste

Flat-leaf parsley or mint, chopped, for garnish

1. Combine the oats and water in a medium saucepan and bring to a boil over high heat, stirring continuously, or until the water is absorbed, about 15 minutes.
2. Divide the oatmeal between 2 bowls and scatter the tomato and cucumber on top. Drizzle with the olive oil and sprinkle with the Parmesan cheese.
3. Season with salt and pepper to taste. Serve garnished with the parsley.

Per Serving

calories: 197| fat: 8.9g | protein: 6.3g | carbs: 23.1g | fiber: 6.4g | sodium: 27mg

Feta and Olive Scrambled Eggs

Prep time: 5 minutes | Cook time: 5 minutes | Serves 2

- 4 large eggs
- 1 tablespoon unsweetened almond milk
- Sea salt and freshly ground pepper, to taste
- 1 tablespoon olive oil
- ¼ cup crumbled feta cheese
- 10 Kalamata olives, pitted and sliced
- Small bunch fresh mint, chopped, for garnish

1. Beat the eggs in a bowl until just combined. Add the milk and a pinch of sea salt and whisk well.
2. Heat a medium nonstick skillet over medium-high heat and add the olive oil.
3. Pour in the egg mixture and stir constantly, or until they just begin to curd and firm up, about 2 minutes. Add the feta cheese and olive slices, and stir until evenly combined. Season to taste with salt and pepper.
4. Divide the mixture between 2 plates and serve garnished with the fresh chopped mint.

Per Serving

calories: 244 | fat: 21.9g | protein: 8.4g | carbs:3.5g | fiber: 0.6g | sodium: 339mg

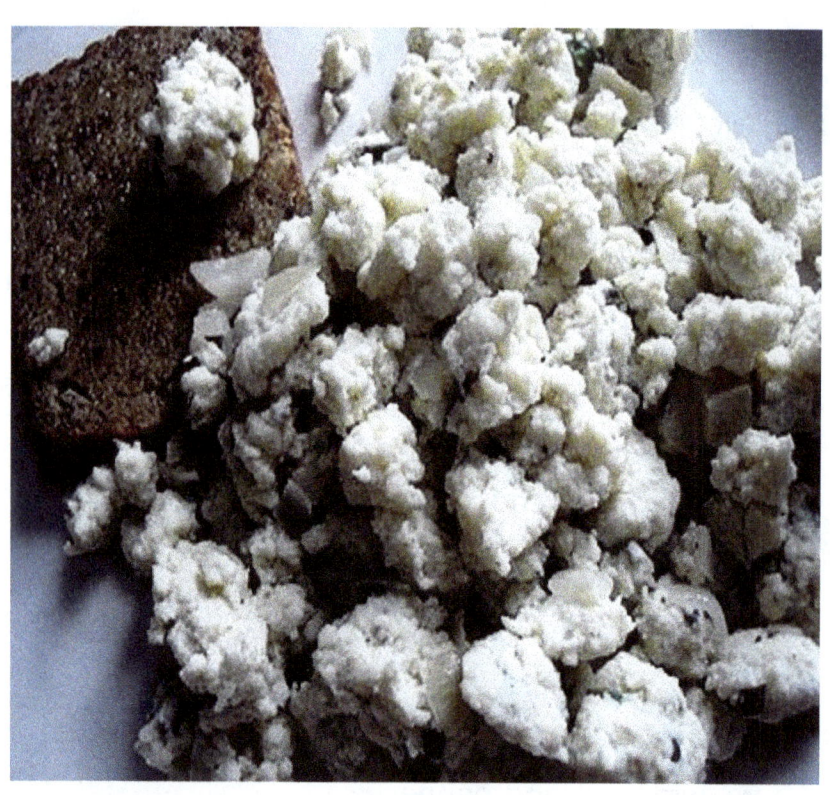

Feta and Spinach Frittata

Prep time: 10 minutes | Cook time: 15 minutes | Serves 2

- 4 large eggs, beaten
- 2 tablespoons fresh chopped herbs, such as rosemary, thyme, oregano, basil or 1 teaspoon dried herbs
- ¼ teaspoon salt
- Freshly ground black pepper, to taste
- 4 tablespoons extra-virgin olive oil, divided
- 1 cup fresh spinach, arugula, kale, or other leafy greens
- 4 ounces (113 g) quartered artichoke hearts, rinsed, drained, and thoroughly dried
- 8 cherry tomatoes, halved
- ½ cup crumbled soft goat cheese

1. Preheat the broiler to Low.
2. In a small bowl, combine the beaten eggs, herbs, salt, and pepper and whisk well with a fork. Set aside.
3. In an ovenproof skillet, heat 2 tablespoons of olive oil over medium heat. Add the spinach, artichoke hearts, and cherry tomatoes and sauté until just wilted, 1 to 2 minutes.

4. Pour in the egg mixture and let it cook undisturbed over medium heat for 3 to 4 minutes, until the eggs begin to set on the bottom.
5. Sprinkle the goat cheese across the top of the egg mixture and transfer the skillet to the oven.
6. Broil for 4 to 5 minutes, or until the frittata is firm in the center and golden brown on top.
7. Remove from the oven and run a rubber spatula around the edge to loosen the sides. Slice the frittata in half and serve drizzled with the remaining 2 tablespoons of olive oil.

Per Serving

calories: 529 | fat: 46.5g | protein: 21.4g | carbs: 7.1g | fiber: 3.1g | sodium: 762mg

Avocado and Egg Toast

Prep time: 5 minutes | Cook time: 8 minutes | Serves 2

2 tablespoons ground flaxseed

½ teaspoon baking powder

2 large eggs, beaten

1 teaspoon salt, plus additional for serving

½ teaspoon freshly ground black pepper, plus additional for serving

½ teaspoon garlic powder, sesame seed, caraway seed, or other dried herbs (optional)

3 tablespoons extra-virgin olive oil, divided

1 medium ripe avocado, peeled, pitted, and sliced

2 tablespoons chopped ripe tomato

1. In a small bowl, combine the flaxseed and baking powder, breaking up any lumps in the baking powder.
2. Add the beaten eggs, salt, pepper, and garlic powder (if desired) and whisk well. Let sit for 2 minutes.
3. In a small nonstick skillet, heat 1 tablespoon of olive oil over medium heat. Pour the egg mixture into the skillet and let cook undisturbed

until the egg begins to set on bottom, 2 to 3 minutes.
4. Using a rubber spatula, scrape down the sides to allow uncooked egg to reach the bottom. Cook for an additional 2 to 3 minutes.
5. Once almost set, flip like a pancake and allow the top to fully cook, another 1 to 2 minutes.
6. Remove from the skillet and allow to cool slightly, then slice into 2 pieces.
7. Top each piece with avocado slices, additional salt and pepper, chopped tomato, and drizzle with the remaining 2 tablespoons of olive oil. Serve immediately.

Per Serving

calories: 297 | fat: 26.1g | protein: 8.9g | carbs: 12.0g | fiber: 7.1g | sodium: 1132mg

Tomato and Egg Breakfast Pizza

Prep time: 5 minutes | Cook time: 15 minutes | Serves 2

2 (6- to 8-inch-long) slices of whole-wheat naan bread

2 tablespoons prepared pesto

1 medium tomato, sliced

2 large eggs

1. Heat a large nonstick skillet over medium-high heat. Place the naan bread in the skillet and let warm for about 2 minutes on each side, or until softened.
2. Spread 1 tablespoon of the pesto on one side of each slice and top with tomato slices.
3. Remove from the skillet and place each one on its own plate.
4. Crack the eggs into the skillet, keeping them separated, and cook until the whites are no longer translucent and the yolk is cooked to desired doneness.
5. Using a spatula, spoon one egg onto each bread slice. Serve warm.

Per Serving

calories: 429 | fat: 16.8g | protein: 18.1g | carbs: 12.0g | fiber: 4.8g | sodium: 682mg

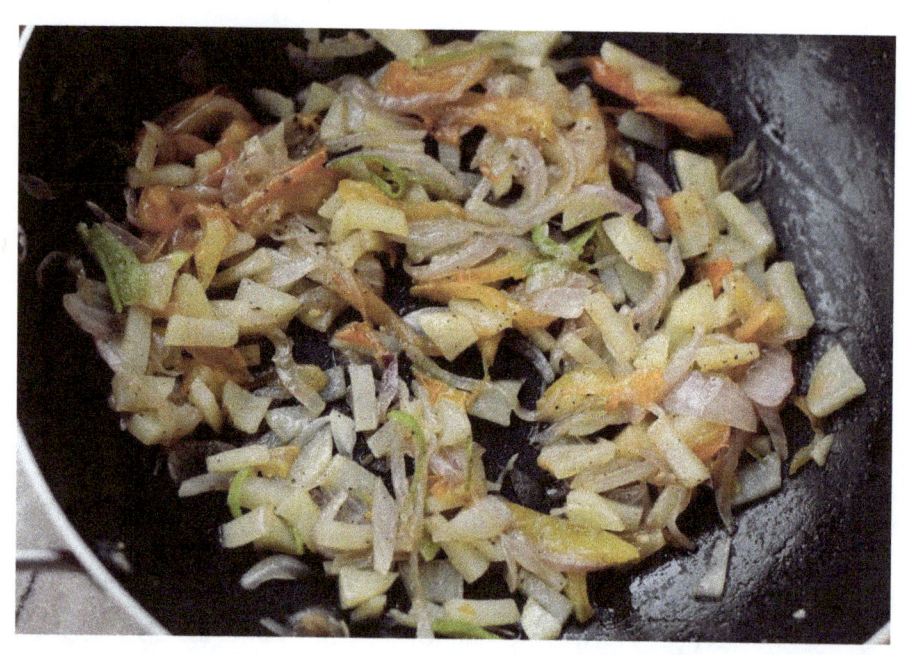

Classic Shakshuka

Prep time: 15 minutes | Cook time: 30 minutes | Serves 2

1 tablespoon olive oil

½ red pepper, diced

½ medium onion, diced

2 small garlic cloves, minced

½ teaspoon smoked paprika

½ teaspoon cumin

Pinch red pepper flakes

1 (14.5-ounce / 411-g) can fire-roasted tomatoes

¼ teaspoon salt

Pinch freshly ground black pepper

1 ounce (28 g) crumbled feta cheese (about ¼ cup)

3 large eggs

3 tablespoons minced fresh parsley

1. Heat the olive oil in a skillet over medium-high heat and add the pepper, onion, and garlic. Sauté until the vegetables start to turn golden.
2. Add the paprika, cumin, and red pepper flakes and stir to toast the spices for about 30 seconds. Add the tomatoes with their juices.
3. Reduce the heat and let the sauce simmer for 10 minutes, or until it starts to thicken. Add the

salt and pepper. Taste the sauce and adjust seasonings as necessary.
4. Scatter the feta cheese on top. Make 3 wells in the sauce and crack one egg into each well.
5. Cover and let the eggs cook for about 7 minutes. Remove the lid and continue cooking for 5 minutes more, or until the yolks are cooked to desired doneness.
6. Garnish with fresh parsley and serve.

Per Serving

calories: 289 | fat: 18.2g | protein: 15.1g | carbs: 18.5g | fiber: 4.9g | sodium: 432mg

Parmesan Oatmeal with Greens

Prep time: 10 minutes | Cook time: 18 minutes | Serves 2

1 tablespoon olive oil

¼ cup minced onion

2 cups greens (arugula, baby spinach, chopped kale, or Swiss chard)

¾ cup gluten-free old-fashioned oats

1½ cups water, or low-sodium chicken stock

2 tablespoons Parmesan cheese

Salt, to taste

Pinch freshly ground black pepper

1. Heat the olive oil in a saucepan over medium-high heat. Add the minced onion and sauté for 2 minutes, or until softened.
2. Add the greens and stir until they begin to wilt. Transfer this mixture to a bowl and set aside.
3. Add the oats to the pan and let them toast for about 2 minutes. Add the water and bring the oats to a boil.
4. Reduce the heat to low, cover, and let the oats cook for 10 minutes, or until the liquid is absorbed and the oats are tender.
5. Stir the Parmesan cheese into the oats, and add the onion and greens back to the pan. Add

additional water if needed, so the oats are creamy and not dry.

6. Stir well and season with salt and black pepper to taste. Serve warm.

Per Serving

calories: 257 | fat: 14.0g | protein: 12.2g | carbs: 30.2g | fiber: 6.1g | sodium: 262mg

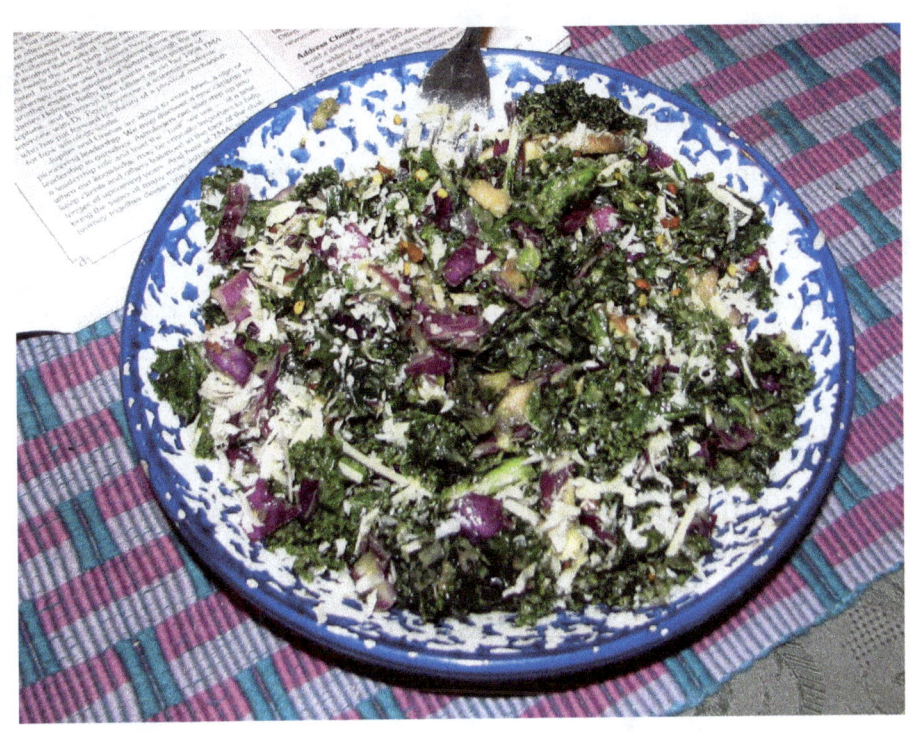

Mediterranean Omelet

Prep time: 8 minutes | Cook time: 15 minutes | Serves 2

2 teaspoons extra-virgin olive oil, divided

1 garlic clove, minced

½ yellow bell pepper, thinly sliced

½ red bell pepper, thinly sliced

¼ cup thinly sliced red onion

2 tablespoons chopped fresh parsley, plus extra for garnish

2 tablespoons chopped fresh basil

½ teaspoon salt

½ teaspoon freshly ground black pepper

4 large eggs, beaten

1. In a large, heavy skillet, heat 1 teaspoon of the olive oil over medium heat. Add the garlic, peppers, and onion to the skillet and sauté, stirring frequently, for 5 minutes.
2. Add the parsley, basil, salt, and pepper, increase the heat to medium-high, and sauté for 2 minutes. Slide the vegetable mixture onto a plate and return the skillet to the heat.
3. Heat the remaining 1 teaspoon of olive oil in the skillet and pour in the beaten eggs, tilting the pan to coat evenly. Cook the eggs just until the

edges are bubbly and all but the center is dry, 3 to 5 minutes.

4. Spoon the vegetable mixture onto one-half of the omelet and use a spatula to fold the empty side over the top. Slide the omelet onto a platter or cutting board.
5. To serve, cut the omelet in half and garnish with extra fresh parsley.

Per Serving

calories: 206 | fat: 14.2g | protein: 13.7g | carbs: 7.2g | fiber: 1.2g | sodium: 729mg

Berry and Nut Parfait

Prep time: 10 minutes | Cook time: 0 minutes | Serves 2

2 cups plain Greek yogurt 1 cup fresh blueberries

2 tablespoons honey ½ cup walnut pieces

1 cup fresh raspberries

1. In a medium bowl, whisk the yogurt and honey. Spoon into 2 serving bowls.
2. Top each with ½ cup blueberries, ½ cup raspberries, and ¼ cup walnut pieces. Serve immediately.

Per Serving

calories: 507 | fat: 23.0g | protein: 24.1g | carbs: 57.0g | fiber: 8.2g | sodium: 172mg

Sides, Salads, and Soups

Pumpkin Soup with Crispy Sage Leaves

Prep time: 15 minutes | Cook time: 10 minutes | Serves 4

- 1 tablespoon olive oil
- 2 garlic cloves, cut into ⅛-inch-thick slices
- 1 onion, chopped
- 2 cups freshly puréed pumpkin
- 4 cups low-sodium vegetable soup
- 2 teaspoons chipotle powder
- 1 teaspoon sea salt
- ½ teaspoon freshly ground black pepper
- ½ cup vegetable oil
- 12 sage leaves, stemmed

1. Heat the olive oil in a stockpot over high heat until shimmering.
2. Add the garlic and onion, then sauté for 5 minutes or until the onion is translucent.
3. Pour in the puréed pumpkin and vegetable soup in the pot, then sprinkle with chipotle powder, salt, and ground black pepper. Stir to mix well.

4. Bring to a boil. Reduce the heat to low and simmer for 5 minutes.
5. Meanwhile, heat the vegetable oil in a nonstick skillet over high heat.
6. Add the sage leaf to the skillet and sauté for a minute or until crispy. Transfer the sage on paper towels to soak the excess oil.
7. Gently pour the soup in three serving bowls, then divide the crispy sage leaves in bowls for garnish. Serve immediately.

Per Serving

calories: 380 | fat: 20.1g | protein: 8.9g | carbs: 45.2g | fiber: 18.0g | sodium: 1364mg

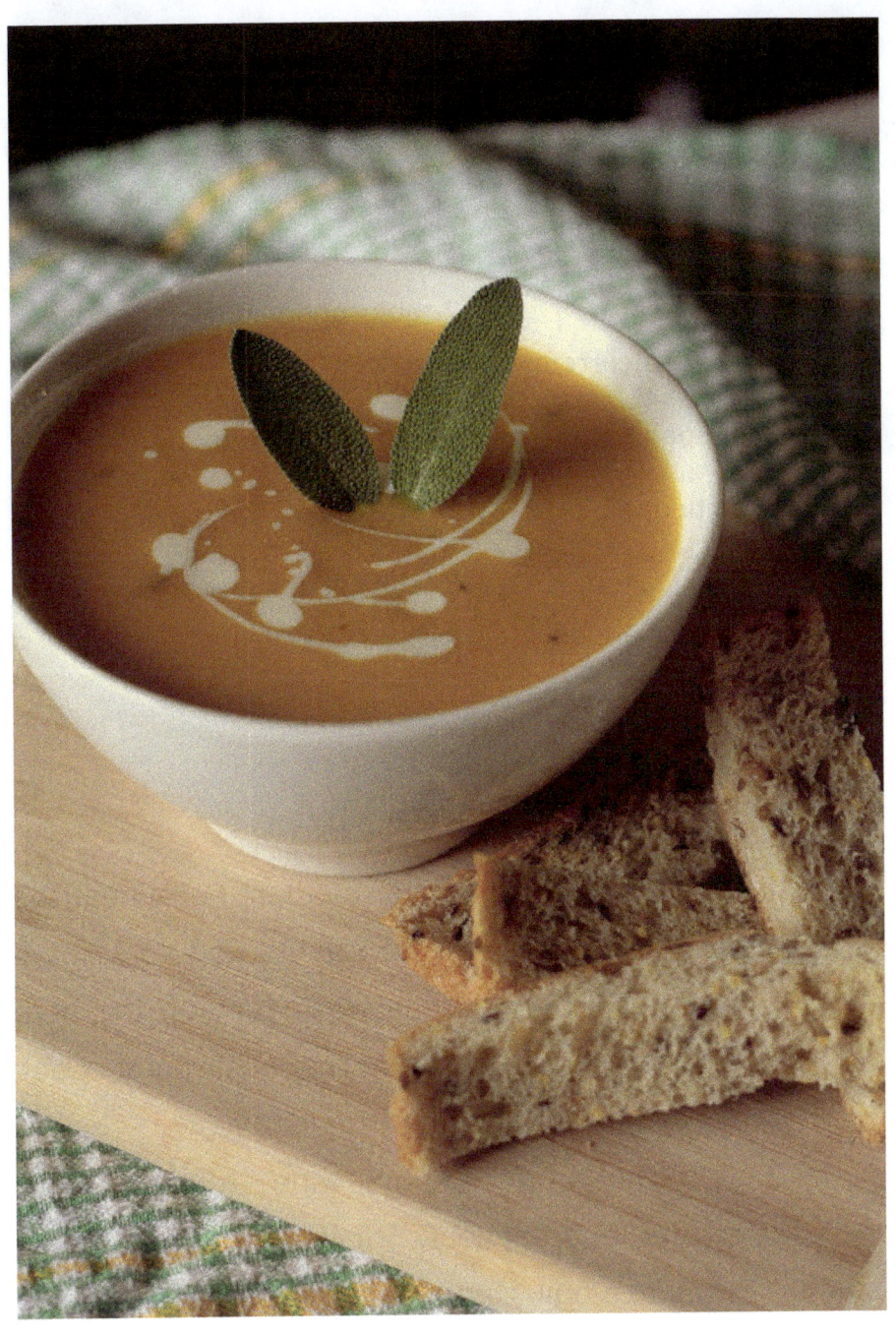

Mushroom Barley Soup

Prep time: 5 minutes | Cook time: 20 to 23 minutes | Serves 6

2 tablespoons extra-virgin olive oil

1 cup chopped carrots

1 cup chopped onion

5½ cups chopped mushrooms

6 cups no-salt-added vegetable broth

1 cup uncooked pearled barley

¼ cup red wine

2 tablespoons tomato paste

4 sprigs fresh thyme or ½ teaspoon dried thyme

1 dried bay leaf

6 tablespoons grated Parmesan cheese

1. In a large stockpot over medium heat, heat the oil. Add the onion and carrots and cook for 5 minutes, stirring frequently. Turn up the heat to medium-high and add the mushrooms. Cook for 3 minutes, stirring frequently.
2. Add the broth, barley, wine, tomato paste, thyme, and bay leaf. Stir, cover, and bring the soup to a boil. Once it's boiling, stir a few times, reduce the heat to medium-low, cover, and

cook for another 12 to 15 minutes, until the barley is cooked through.

3. Remove the bay leaf and serve the soup in bowls with 1 tablespoon of cheese sprinkled on top of each.

Per Serving

calories: 195 | fat: 4.0g | protein: 7.0g | carbs: 34.0g | fiber: 6.0g | sodium: 173mg

Paella Soup

Prep time: 6 minutes | Cook time: 24 minutes | Serves 6

- 2 tablespoons extra-virgin olive oil
- 1 cup chopped onion
- 1½ cups coarsely chopped green bell pepper
- 1½ cups coarsely chopped red bell pepper
- 2 garlic cloves, chopped
- 1 teaspoon ground turmeric
- 1 teaspoon dried thyme
- 2 teaspoons smoked paprika
- 2½ cups uncooked instant brown rice
- 2 cups low-sodium or no-salt-added chicken broth
- 2½ cups water
- 1 cup frozen green peas, thawed
- 1 (28-ounce / 794-g) can low-sodium or no-salt-added crushed tomatoes
- 1 pound (454 g) fresh raw medium shrimp, shells and tails removed

1. In a large stockpot over medium-high heat, heat the oil. Add the onion, bell peppers, and

garlic. Cook for 8 minutes, stirring occasionally. Add the turmeric, thyme, and smoked paprika, and cook for 2 minutes more, stirring often. Stir in the rice, broth, and water. Bring to a boil over high heat. Cover, reduce the heat to medium-low, and cook for 10 minutes.

2. Stir the peas, tomatoes, and shrimp into the soup. Cook for 4 minutes, until the shrimp is cooked, turning from gray to pink and white. The soup will be very thick, almost like stew, when ready to serve.
3. Ladle the soup into bowls and serve hot.

Per Serving

calories: 431 | fat: 5.7g | protein: 26.0g | carbs: 69.1g | fiber: 7.4g | sodium: 203mg

Parmesan Roasted Red Potatoes

Prep time: 10 minutes | Cook time: 55 minutes | Serves 2

12 ounces (340 g) red potatoes (3 to 4 small potatoes), scrubbed and diced into 1-inch pieces

1 tablespoon olive oil

½ teaspoon garlic powder

¼ teaspoon salt

1 tablespoon grated Parmesan cheese

1 teaspoon minced fresh rosemary (from 1 sprig)

1. Preheat the oven to 425ºF (220ºC). Line a baking sheet with parchment paper.
2. In a mixing bowl, combine the potatoes, olive oil, garlic powder, and salt. Toss well to coat.
3. Lay the potatoes on the parchment paper and roast for 10 minutes. Flip the potatoes over and roast for another 10 minutes.
4. Check the potatoes to make sure they are golden brown on the top and bottom. Toss them again, turn the heat down to 350ºF (180ºC), and roast for 30 minutes more.
5. When the potatoes are golden brown, scatter the Parmesan cheese over them and toss again.

Return to the oven for 3 minutes to melt the cheese.
6. Remove from the oven and sprinkle with the fresh rosemary before serving.

Per Serving

calories: 200 | fat: 8.2g | protein: 5.1g | carbs: 30.0g | fiber: 3.2g | sodium: 332mg

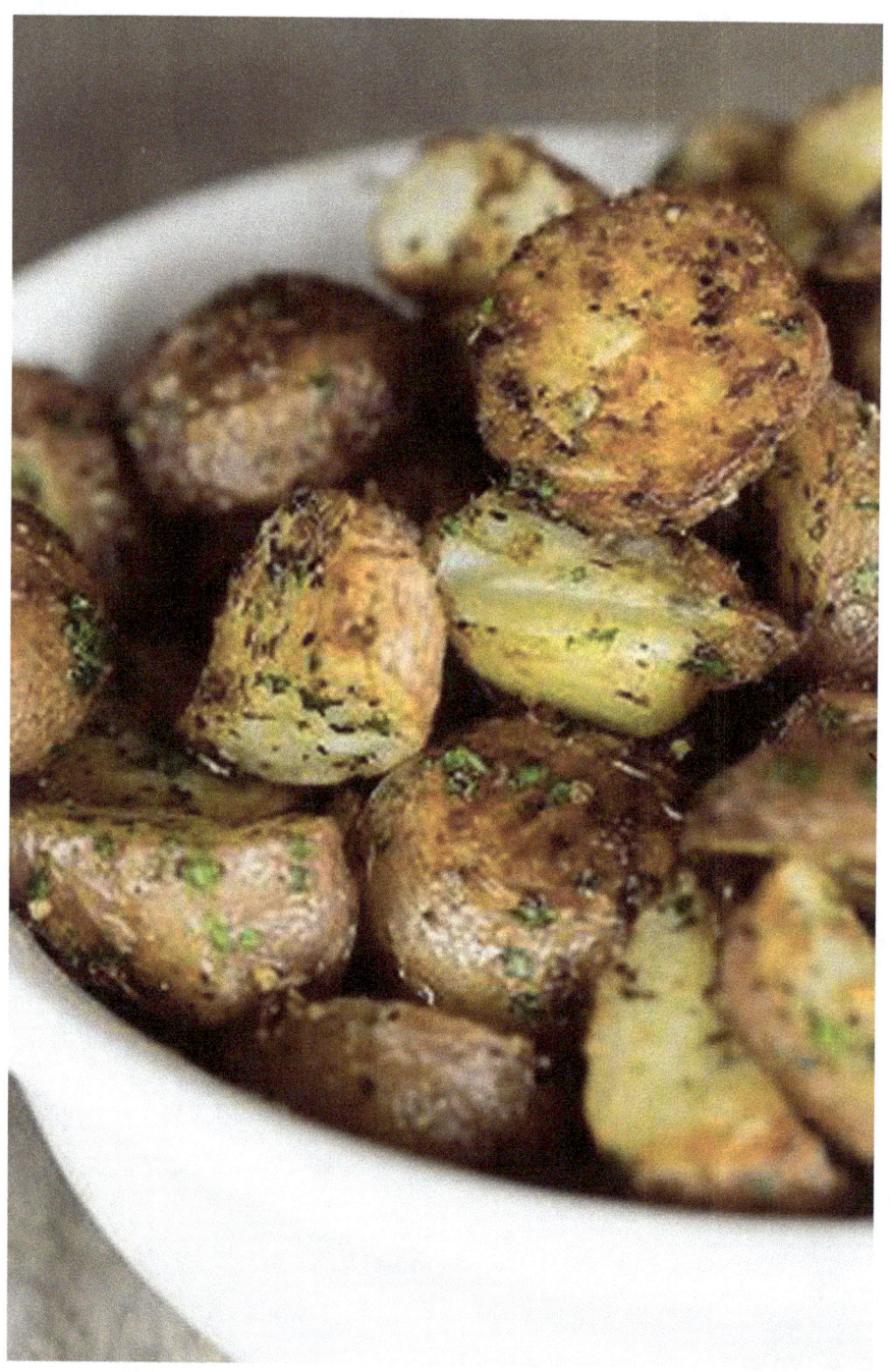

Garlic Wilted Greens

Prep time: 10 minutes | Cook time: 5 minutes | Serves 2

- 1 tablespoon olive oil
- 2 garlic cloves, minced
- 3 cups sliced greens (spinach, chard, beet greens, dandelion greens, or a combination)
- Pinch salt
- Pinch red pepper flakes (or more to taste)

1. Heat the olive oil in a skillet over medium-high heat.
2. Add garlic and sauté for 30 seconds, or just until fragrant.
3. Add the greens, salt, and pepper flakes and stir to combine. Let the greens wilt, but do not overcook.
4. Remove from the skillet and serve on a plate.

Per Serving

calories: 93 | fat: 6.8g | protein: 1.2g | carbs: 7.3g | fiber: 3.1g | sodium: 112mg

Sautéed Kale with Olives

Prep time: 10 minutes | Cook time: 10 minutes | Serves 2

1 bunch kale, leaves chopped and stems minced

½ cup celery leaves, roughly chopped, or additional parsley

½ bunch flat-leaf parsley, stems and leaves roughly chopped

4 garlic cloves, chopped

2 teaspoons olive oil

¼ cup pitted Kalamata olives, chopped

Grated zest and juice of 1 lemon

Salt and pepper, to taste

1. Place the kale, celery leaves, parsley, and garlic in a steamer basket set over a medium saucepan. Steam over medium-high heat, covered, for 15 minutes. Remove from the heat and squeeze out any excess moisture.
2. Place a large skillet over medium heat. Add the oil, then add the kale mixture to the skillet. Cook, stirring often, for 5 minutes.
3. Remove from the heat and add the olives and lemon zest and juice. Season with salt and pepper and serve.

Per Serving

calories: 86 | fat: 6.4g | protein: 1.8g | carbs: 7.5g | fiber: 2.1g | sodium: 276mg

Balsamic Brussels Sprouts and Delicata Squash

Prep time: 10 minutes | Cook time: 30 minutes | Serves 2

½ pound (227 g) Brussels sprouts, ends trimmed and outer leaves removed

1 medium delicata squash, halved lengthwise, seeded, and cut into 1-inch pieces

1 cup fresh cranberries

2 teaspoons olive oil

Salt and freshly ground black pepper, to taste

½ cup balsamic vinegar

2 tablespoons roasted pumpkin seeds

2 tablespoons fresh pomegranate arils (seeds)

1. Preheat oven to 400ºF (205ºC). Line a sheet pan with parchment paper.
2. Combine the Brussels sprouts, squash, and cranberries in a large bowl. Drizzle with olive oil, and season lightly with salt and pepper. Toss well to coat and arrange in a single layer on the sheet pan.

3. Roast in the preheated oven for 30 minutes, turning vegetables halfway through, or until Brussels sprouts turn brown and crisp in spots.
4. Meanwhile, make the balsamic glaze by simmering the vinegar for 10 to 12 minutes, or until mixture has reduced to about ¼ cup and turns a syrupy consistency.
5. Remove the vegetables from the oven, drizzle with balsamic syrup, and sprinkle with pumpkin seeds and pomegranate arils before serving.

Per Serving

calories: 203 | fat: 6.8g | protein: 6.2g | carbs: 22.0g | fiber: 8.2g | sodium: 32mg

Green Beans with Tahini-Lemon Sauce

Prep time: 5 minutes | Cook time: 10 minutes | Serves 2

1 pound (454 g) green beans, washed and trimmed

2 tablespoons tahini

1 garlic clove, minced

Grated zest and juice of 1 lemon

Salt and black pepper, to taste

1 teaspoon toasted black or white sesame seeds (optional)

1. Steam the beans in a medium saucepan fitted with a steamer basket (or by adding ¼ cup water to a covered saucepan) over medium-high heat. Drain, reserving the cooking water.
2. Mix the tahini, garlic, lemon zest and juice, and salt and pepper to taste. Use the reserved cooking water to thin the sauce as desired.
3. Toss the green beans with the sauce and garnish with the sesame seeds, if desired. Serve immediately.

Per Serving

calories: 188 | fat: 8.4g | protein: 7.2g | carbs: 22.2g | fiber: 7.9g | sodium: 200mg

Mixed Salad With Balsamic Honey Dressing

Prep time: 15 minutes | Cook time: 0 minutes | Serves 2

Dressing:

¼ cup balsamic vinegar

¼ cup olive oil

1 tablespoon honey

1 teaspoon Dijon mustard

¼ teaspoon garlic powder

¼ teaspoon salt, or more to taste

Pinch freshly ground black pepper

Salad:

4 cups chopped red leaf lettuce

½ cup cherry or grape tomatoes, halved

½ English cucumber, sliced in quarters lengthwise and then cut into bite-size pieces

Any combination fresh, torn herbs (parsley, oregano, basil, or chives)

1 tablespoon roasted sunflower seeds

Make the Dressing

1. Combine the vinegar, olive oil, honey, mustard, garlic powder, salt, and pepper in a jar with a lid. Shake well.

Make the Salad

2. In a large bowl, combine the lettuce, tomatoes, cucumber, and herbs. Toss well.
3. Pour all or as much dressing as desired over the tossed salad and toss again to coat the salad with dressing.
4. Top with the sunflower seeds before serving.

Per Serving

calories: 337 | fat: 26.1g | protein: 4.2g | carbs: 22.2g | fiber: 3.1g | sodium: 172mg

Arugula and Fig Salad

Prep time: 15 minutes | Cook time: 0 minutes | Serves 2

- 3 cups arugula
- 4 fresh, ripe figs (or 4 to 6 dried figs), stemmed and sliced
- 2 tablespoons olive oil
- ¼ cup lightly toasted pecan halves
- 2 tablespoons crumbled blue cheese
- 1 to 2 tablespoons balsamic glaze

1. Toss the arugula and figs with the olive oil in a large bowl until evenly coated.
2. Add the pecans and blue cheese to the bowl. Toss the salad lightly.
3. Drizzle with the balsamic glaze and serve immediately.

Per Serving

calories: 517 | fat: 36.2g | protein: 18.9g | carbs: 30.2g | fiber: 6.1g | sodium: 481mg

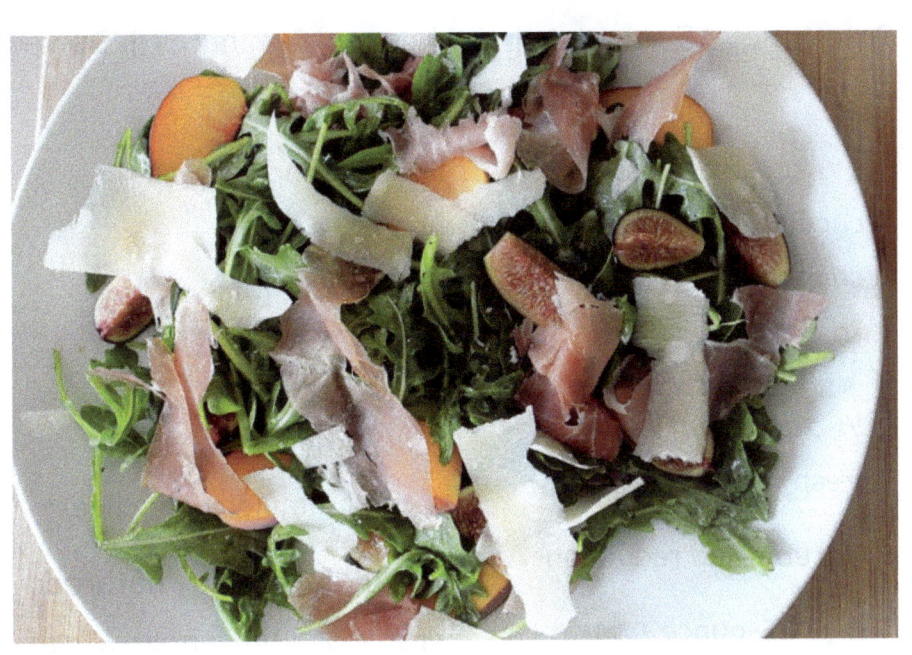

Sandwiches, Pizzas, and Wraps

Mediterranean Greek Salad Wraps

Prep time: 15 minutes | Cook time: 0 minutes | Serves 4

1½ cups seedless cucumber, peeled and chopped

1 cup chopped tomato

½ cup finely chopped fresh mint

¼ cup diced red onion

1 (2.25-ounce / 64-g) can sliced black olives, drained

2 tablespoons extra-virgin olive oil

1 tablespoon red wine vinegar

¼ teaspoon kosher salt

¼ teaspoon freshly ground black pepper

½ cup crumbled goat cheese

4 whole-wheat flatbread wraps or soft whole-wheat tortillas

1. In a large bowl, stir together the cucumber, tomato, mint, onion and olives.

2. In a small bowl, whisk together the oil, vinegar, salt, and pepper. Spread the dressing over the salad. Toss gently to combine.
3. On a clean work surface, lay the wraps. Divide the goat cheese evenly among the wraps. Scoop a quarter of the salad filling down the center of each wrap.
4. Fold up each wrap: Start by folding up the bottom, then fold one side over and fold the other side over the top. Repeat with the remaining wraps.
5. Serve immediately.

Per Serving

calories: 225 | fat: 12.0g | protein: 12.0g | carbs: 18.0g | fiber: 4.0g | sodium: 349mg

Salmon Salad Wraps

Prep time: 10 minutes | Cook time: 0 minutes | Serves 6

- 1 pound (454 g) salmon fillets, cooked and flaked
- ½ cup diced carrots
- ½ cup diced celery
- 3 tablespoons diced red onion
- 3 tablespoons chopped fresh dill
- 2 tablespoons capers
- 1½ tablespoons extra-virgin olive oil
- 1 tablespoon aged balsamic vinegar
- ¼ teaspoon kosher or sea salt
- ½ teaspoon freshly ground black pepper
- 4 whole-wheat flatbread wraps or soft whole-wheat tortillas

1. In a large bowl, stir together all the ingredients, except for the wraps.
2. On a clean work surface, lay the wraps. Divide the salmon mixture evenly among the wraps. Fold up the bottom of the wraps, then roll up the wrap.
3. Serve immediately.

Per Serving

calories: 194 | fat: 8.0g | protein: 18.0g | carbs: 13.0g | fiber: 3.0g | sodium: 536mg

Baked Parmesan Chicken Wraps

Prep time: 10 minutes | Cook time: 18 minutes | Serves 6

1 pound (454 g) boneless, skinless chicken breasts

1 large egg

¼ cup unsweetened almond milk

⅔ cup whole-wheat bread crumbs

½ cup grated Parmesan cheese

¾ teaspoon garlic powder, divided

1 cup canned low-sodium or no-salt-added crushed tomatoes

1 teaspoon dried oregano

6 (8-inch) whole-wheat tortillas, or whole-grain spinach wraps

1 cup fresh Mozzarella cheese, sliced

1½ cups loosely packed fresh flat-leaf (Italian) parsley, chopped

Cooking spray

1. Preheat the oven to 425ºF (220ºC). Line a large, rimmed baking sheet with aluminum foil. Place a wire rack on the aluminum foil, and spritz the rack with nonstick cooking spray. Set aside.

2. Place the chicken breasts into a large plastic bag. With a rolling pin, pound the chicken so it is evenly flattened, about ¼ inch thick. Slice the chicken into six portions.
3. In a bowl, whisk together the egg and milk. In another bowl, stir together the bread crumbs, Parmesan cheese and ½ teaspoon of the garlic powder.
4. Dredge each chicken breast portion into the egg mixture, and then into the Parmesan crumb mixture, pressing the crumbs into the chicken so they stick. Arrange the chicken on the prepared wire rack.
5. Bake in the preheated oven for 15 to 18 minutes, or until the internal temperature of the chicken reads 165ºF (74ºC) on a meat thermometer and any juices run clear.
6. Transfer the chicken to a cutting board, and cut each portion diagonally into ½-inch pieces.
7. In a small, microwave-safe bowl, stir together the tomatoes, oregano, and the remaining ¼ teaspoon of the garlic powder. Cover the bowl with a paper towel and microwave for about 1 minute on high, until very hot. Set aside.

8. Wrap the tortillas in a damp paper towel and microwave for 30 to 45 seconds on high, or until warmed through.
9. Assemble the wraps: Divide the chicken slices evenly among the six tortillas and top with the sliced Mozzarella cheese. Spread 1 tablespoon of the warm tomato sauce over the cheese on each tortilla, and top each with about ¼ cup of the parsley.
10. Wrap the tortilla: Fold up the bottom of the tortilla, then fold one side over and fold the other side over the top.
11. Serve the wraps warm with the remaining sauce for dipping.

Per Serving

calories: 358 | fat: 12.0g | protein: 21.0g | carbs: 41.0g | fiber: 7.0g | sodium: 755mg

Eggplant, Spinach, and Feta Sandwiches

Prep time: 10 minutes | Cook time: 6 to 8 minutes | Serves 2

1 medium eggplant, sliced into ½-inch-thick slices

2 tablespoons olive oil

Sea salt and freshly ground pepper, to taste

5 to 6 tablespoons hummus

4 slices whole-wheat bread, toasted

1 cup baby spinach leaves

2 ounces (57 g) feta cheese, softened

1. Preheat the grill to medium-high heat.
2. Salt both sides of the sliced eggplant, and let sit for 20 minutes to draw out the bitter juices.
3. Rinse the eggplant and pat dry with a paper towel.
4. Brush the eggplant slices with olive oil and season with sea salt and freshly ground pepper to taste.
5. Grill the eggplant until lightly charred on both sides but still slightly firm in the middle, about 3 to 4 minutes per side.

6. Spread the hummus on the bread slices and top with the spinach leaves, feta cheese, and grilled eggplant. Top with the other slice of bread and serve immediately.

Per Serving

calories: 493 | fat: 25.3g | protein: 17.1g | carbs: 50.9g | fiber: 14.7g | sodium: 789mg

Grilled Caesar Salad Sandwiches

Prep time: 5 minutes | Cook time: 5 minutes | Serves 2

¾ cup olive oil, divided

2 romaine lettuce hearts, left intact

3 to 4 anchovy fillets

Juice of 1 lemon

2 to 3 cloves garlic, peeled

1 teaspoon Dijon mustard

¼ teaspoon Worcestershire sauce

Sea salt and freshly ground pepper, to taste

2 slices whole-wheat bread, toasted

Freshly grated Parmesan cheese, for serving

1. Preheat the grill to medium-high heat and oil the grates.
2. On a cutting board, drizzle the lettuce with 1 to 2 tablespoons of olive oil and place on the grates.
3. Grill for 5 minutes, turning until lettuce is slightly charred on all sides. Let lettuce cool enough to handle.
4. In a food processor, combine the remaining olive oil with the anchovies, lemon juice, garlic, mustard, and Worcestershire sauce.

5. Pulse the ingredients until you have a smooth emulsion. Season with sea salt and freshly ground pepper to taste. Chop the lettuce in half and place on the bread.
6. Drizzle with the dressing and serve with a sprinkle of Parmesan cheese.

Per Serving

calories: 949 | fat: 85.6g | protein: 12.9g | carbs: 34.1g | fiber: 13.9g | sodium: 786mg

Green Veggie Sandwiches

Prep time: 20 minutes | Cook time: 0 minutes | Serves 2

Spread:

1 (15-ounce / 425-g) can cannellini beans, drained and rinsed

1/2 cup packed fresh basil leaves

1/2 cup packed fresh parsley

1/2 cup chopped fresh chives

2 garlic cloves, chopped

Zest and juice of ½ lemon

1 tablespoon apple cider vinegar

Sandwiches:

4 whole-grain bread slices, toasted

8 English cucumber slices

1 large beefsteak tomato, cut into slices

1 large avocado, halved, pitted, and cut into slices

1 small yellow bell pepper, cut into slices

2 handfuls broccoli sprouts

2 handfuls fresh spinach

Make the Spread

1. In a food processor, combine the cannellini beans, basil, parsley, chives, garlic, lemon zest and juice, and vinegar. Pulse a few times, scrape down the sides, and purée until smooth. You may need to scrape down the sides again to incorporate all the basil and parsley.

Refrigerate for at least 1 hour to allow the flavors to blend.

1. Assemble the Sandwiches
2. Build your sandwiches by spreading several tablespoons of spread on each slice of bread. Layer two slices of bread with the cucumber, tomato, avocado, bell pepper, broccoli sprouts, and spinach. Top with the remaining bread slices and press down lightly.
3. Serve immediately.

Per Serving

calories: 617 | fat: 21.1g | protein: 28.1g | carbs: 86.1g | fiber: 25.6g | sodium: 593mg

Pizza Pockets

Prep time: 10 minutes | Cook time: 0 minutes | Serves 2

- ½ cup tomato sauce
- ½ teaspoon oregano
- ½ teaspoon garlic powder
- ½ cup chopped black olives
- 2 canned artichoke hearts, drained and chopped
- 2 ounces (57 g) pepperoni, chopped
- ½ cup shredded Mozzarella cheese
- 1 whole-wheat pita, halved

1. In a medium bowl, stir together the tomato sauce, oregano, and garlic powder.
2. Add the olives, artichoke hearts, pepperoni, and cheese. Stir to mix.
3. Spoon the mixture into the pita halves and serve.

Per Serving

calories: 375 | fat: 23.5g | protein: 17.1g | carbs: 27.1g | fiber: 6.1g | sodium: 1080mg

Mushroom-Pesto Baked Pizza

Prep time: 5 minutes | Cook time: 15 minutes | Serves 2

1 teaspoon extra-virgin olive oil

½ cup sliced mushrooms

½ red onion, sliced

Salt and freshly ground black pepper

¼ cup store-bought pesto sauce

2 whole-wheat flatbreads

¼ cup shredded Mozzarella cheese

1. Preheat the oven to 350°F (180°C).
2. In a small skillet, heat the oil over medium heat. Add the mushrooms and onion, and season with salt and pepper. Sauté for 3 to 5 minutes until the onion and mushrooms begin to soften.
3. Spread 2 tablespoons of pesto on each flatbread.
4. Divide the mushroom-onion mixture between the two flatbreads. Top each with 2 tablespoons of cheese.
5. Place the flatbreads on a baking sheet and bake for 10 to 12 minutes until the cheese is melted and bubbly. Serve warm.

Per Serving

calories: 348 | fat: 23.5g | protein: 14.2g | carbs: 28.1g | fiber: 7.1g | sodium: 792mg

Tuna and Hummus Wraps

Prep time: 10 minutes | Cook time: 0 minutes | Serves 2

Hummus:

1 cup from 1 (15-ounce / 425-g) can low-sodium chickpeas, drained and rinsed

2 tablespoons tahini

1 tablespoon extra-virgin olive oil

1 garlic clove

Juice of ½ lemon

¼ teaspoon salt

2 tablespoons water

Wraps:

4 large lettuce leaves

1 (5-ounce / 142-g) can chunk light tuna packed in water, drained

1 red bell pepper, seeded and cut into strips

1 cucumber, sliced

Make the Hummus

1. In a blender jar, combine the chickpeas, tahini, olive oil, garlic, lemon juice, salt, and water. Process until smooth. Taste and adjust with additional lemon juice or salt, as needed.

Make the Wraps

2. On each lettuce leaf, spread 1 tablespoon of hummus, and divide the tuna among the

leaves. Top each with several strips of red pepper and cucumber slices.
3. Roll up the lettuce leaves, folding in the two shorter sides and rolling away from you, like a burrito. Serve immediately.

Per Serving

calories: 192 | fat: 5.1g | protein: 26.1g | carbs: 15.1g | fiber: 4.1g | sodium: 352mg

Chickpea Lettuce Wraps

Prep time: 15 minutes | Cook time: 0 minutes | Serves 2

1 (15-ounce / 425-g) can chickpeas, drained and rinsed well

1 celery stalk, diced

½ shallot, minced

1 green apple, cored and diced

3 tablespoons tahini (sesame paste)

2 teaspoons freshly squeezed lemon juice

1 teaspoon raw honey

1 teaspoon Dijon mustard Dash salt

Filtered water, to thin

4 romaine lettuce leaves

1. In a medium bowl, stir together the chickpeas, celery, shallot, apple, tahini, lemon juice, honey, mustard, and salt. If needed, add some water to thin the mixture.
2. Place the romaine lettuce leaves on a plate. Fill each with the chickpea filling, using it all. Wrap the leaves around the filling. Serve immediately.

Per Serving

calories: 397 | fat: 15.1g | protein: 15.1g | carbs: 53.1g | fiber: 15.3g | sodium: 409mg

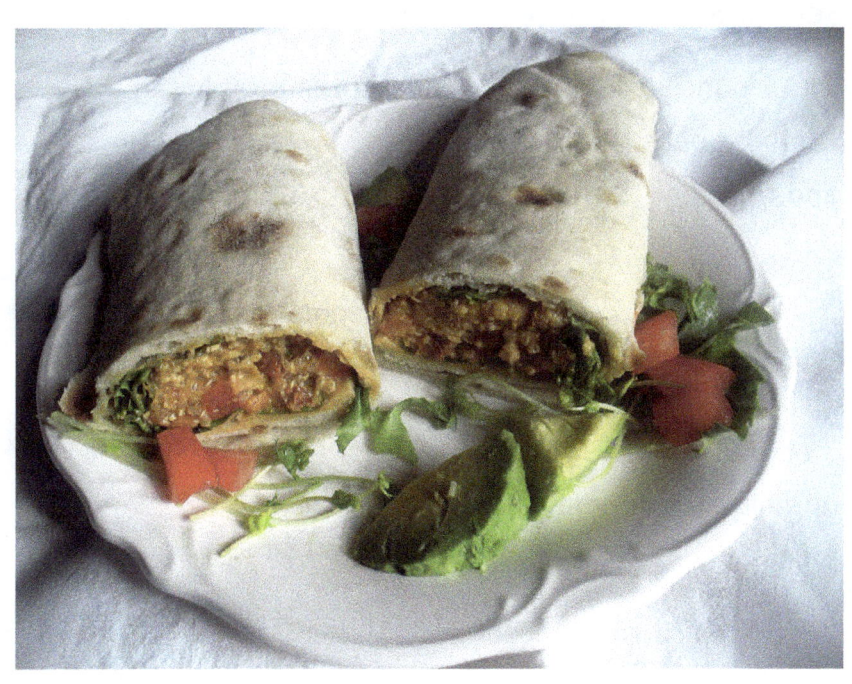

Beans, Grains, and Pastas

Minestrone Chickpeas and Macaroni Casserole

Prep time: 20 minutes | Cook time: 7 hours 20 minutes | Serves 5

- 1 (15-ounce / 425-g) can chickpeas, drained and rinsed
- 1 (28-ounce / 794-g) can diced tomatoes, with the juice
- 1 (6-ounce / 170-g) can no-salt-added tomato paste
- 3 medium carrots, sliced
- 3 cloves garlic, minced
- 1 medium yellow onion, chopped
- 1 cup low-sodium vegetable soup
- 1 teaspoon dried oregano
- 2 teaspoons maple syrup
- ½ teaspoon sea salt
- ¼ teaspoon ground black pepper
- ½ pound (227-g) fresh green beans, trimmed and cut into bite-size pieces
- 1 cup macaroni pasta
- 2 ounces (57 g) Parmesan cheese, grated

½ teaspoon dried rosemary

1. Except for the green beans, pasta, and Parmesan cheese, combine all the ingredients in the slow cooker and stir to mix well.
2. Put the slow cooker lid on and cook on low for 7 hours.
3. Fold in the pasta and green beans. Put the lid on and cook on high for 20 minutes or until the vegetable are soft and the pasta is al dente.
4. Pour them in a large serving bowl and spread with Parmesan cheese before serving.

Per Serving

calories: 349 | fat: 6.7g | protein: 16.5g | carbs: 59.9g | fiber: 12.9g | sodium: 937mg

Turkish Canned Pinto Bean Salad

Prep time: 10 minutes | Cook time: 3 minutes | Serves 4 to 6

¼ cup extra-virgin olive oil, divided

3 garlic cloves, lightly crushed and peeled

2 (15-ounce / 425-g) cans pinto beans, rinsed 2 cups plus

1 tablespoon water

Salt and pepper, to taste

¼ cup tahini

3 tablespoons lemon juice

1 tablespoon ground dried Aleppo pepper, plus extra for serving

8 ounces (227 g) cherry tomatoes, halved

¼ red onion, sliced thinly

½ cup fresh parsley leaves

2 hard-cooked large eggs, quartered

1 tablespoon toasted sesame seeds

1. Add 1 tablespoon of the olive oil and garlic to a medium saucepan over medium heat. Cook for about 3 minutes, stirring constantly, or until the garlic turns golden but not brown.
2. Add the beans, 2 cups of the water and 1 teaspoon salt and bring to a simmer. Remove from the heat, cover and let sit for 20 minutes. Drain the beans and discard the garlic.

Garlic and Parsley Chickpeas

Prep time: 10 minutes | Cook time: 18 to 20 minutes | Serves 4 to 6

¼ cup extra-virgin olive oil, divided

4 garlic cloves, sliced thinly

⅛ teaspoon red pepper flakes

1 onion, chopped finely

¼ teaspoon salt, plus more to taste

Black pepper, to taste

2 (15-ounce / 425-g) cans chickpeas, rinsed

1 cup vegetable broth

2 tablespoons minced fresh parsley

2 teaspoons lemon juice

1. Add 3 tablespoons of the olive oil, garlic, and pepper flakes to a skillet over medium heat. Cook for about 3 minutes, stirring constantly, or until the garlic turns golden but not brown.
2. Stir in the onion and ¼ teaspoon salt and cook for 5 to 7 minutes, or until softened and lightly browned.
3. Add the chickpeas and broth to the skillet and bring to a simmer. Reduce the heat to medium-low, cover, and cook for about 7 minutes, or

until the chickpeas are cooked through and flavors meld.
4. Uncover, increase the heat to high and continue to cook for about 3 minutes more, or until nearly all liquid has evaporated.
5. Turn off the heat, stir in the parsley and lemon juice. Season to taste with salt and pepper and drizzle with remaining 1 tablespoon of the olive oil.
6. Serve warm.

Per Serving

calories: 220 | fat: 11.4g | protein: 6.5g | carbs: 24.6g | fiber: 6.0g | sodium: 467mg

Black-Eyed Peas Salad with Walnuts

Prep time: 10 minutes | Cook time: 0 minutes | Serves 4 to 6

3 tablespoons extra-virgin olive oil

3 tablespoons dukkah, divided

2 tablespoons lemon juice

2 tablespoons pomegranate molasses

¼ teaspoon salt, or more to taste

⅛ teaspoon pepper, or more to taste

2 (15-ounce / 425-g) cans black-eyed peas, rinsed

½ cup pomegranate seeds

½ cup minced fresh parsley

½ cup walnuts, toasted and chopped

4 scallions, sliced thinly

1. In a large bowl, whisk together the olive oil, 2 tablespoons of the dukkah, lemon juice, pomegranate molasses, salt and pepper.
2. Stir in the remaining ingredients. Season with salt and pepper.
3. Sprinkle with the remaining 1 tablespoon of the dukkah before serving.

Per Serving

calories: 155 | fat: 11.5g | protein: 2.0g | carbs: 12.5g | fiber: 2.1g | sodium: 105mg

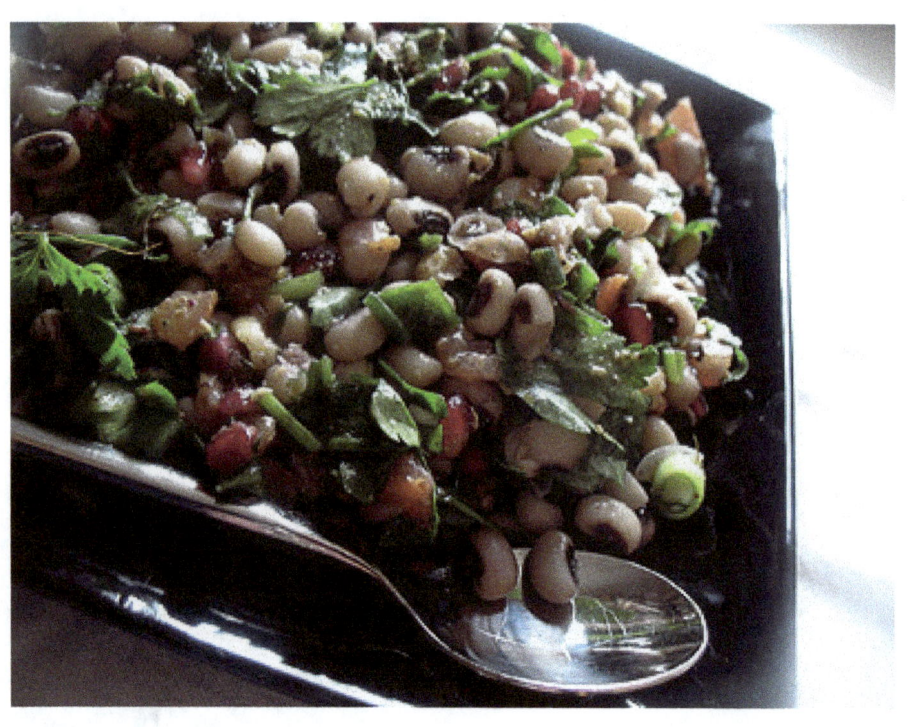

Mashed Beans with Cumin

Prep time: 10 minutes | Cook time: 10 to 12 minutes | Serves 4 to 6

1 tablespoon extra-virgin olive oil, plus extra for serving

4 garlic cloves, minced

1 teaspoon ground cumin

2 (15-ounce / 425-g) cans fava beans

3 tablespoons tahini

2 tablespoons lemon juice, plus lemon wedges for serving

Salt and pepper, to taste

1 tomato, cored and cut into ½-inch pieces

1 small onion, chopped finely

2 hard-cooked large eggs, chopped

2 tablespoons minced fresh parsley

1. Add the olive oil, garlic and cumin to a medium saucepan over medium heat. Cook for about 2 minutes, or until fragrant.
2. Stir in the beans with their liquid and tahini. Bring to a simmer and cook for 8 to 10 minutes, or until the liquid thickens slightly.

3. Turn off the heat, mash the beans to a coarse consistency with a potato masher. Stir in the lemon juice and 1 teaspoon pepper. Season with salt and pepper.
4. Transfer the mashed beans to a serving dish. Top with the tomato, onion, eggs and parsley. Drizzle with the extra olive oil.
5. Serve with the lemon wedges.

Per Serving

calories: 125 | fat: 8.6g | protein: 4.9g | carbs: 9.1g | fiber: 2.9g | sodium: 131mg

3. In a large bowl, whisk together the remaining 3 tablespoons of the oil, tahini, lemon juice, Aleppo, the remaining 1 tablespoon of the water and ¼ teaspoon salt. Stir in the beans, tomatoes, onion and parsley. Season with salt and pepper to taste.
4. Transfer to a serving platter and top with the eggs. Sprinkle with the sesame seeds and extra Aleppo before serving.

Per Serving

calories: 402 | fat: 18.9g | protein: 16.2g | carbs: 44.4g | fiber: 11.2g | sodium: 456mg

Fava and Garbanzo Bean Ful

Prep time: 10 minutes | Cook time: 10 minutes | Serves 6

1 (15-ounce / 425-g) can fava beans, rinsed and drained

1 (1-pound / 454-g) can garbanzo beans, rinsed and drained

3 cups water

½ cup lemon juice

3 cloves garlic, peeled and minced

1 teaspoon salt

3 tablespoons extra-virgin olive oil

1. In a pot over medium heat, cook the beans and water for 10 minutes.
2. Drain the beans and transfer to a bowl. Reserve 1 cup of the liquid from the cooked beans.
3. Add the reserved liquid, lemon juice, minced garlic and salt to the bowl with the beans. Mix to combine well. Using a potato masher, mash up about half the beans in the bowl.
4. Give the mixture one more stir to make sure the beans are evenly mixed.
5. Drizzle with the olive oil and serve.

Per Serving

calories: 199 | fat: 9.0g | protein: 10.0g | carbs: 25.0g | fiber: 9.0g | sodium: 395mg

Triple-Green Pasta with Cheese

Prep time: 5 minutes | Cook time: 14 to 16 minutes | Serves 4

8 ounces (227 g) uncooked penne
1 tablespoon extra-virgin olive oil
2 garlic cloves, minced
¼ teaspoon crushed red pepper
2 cups chopped fresh flat-leaf parsley, including stems
5 cups loosely packed baby spinach
¼ teaspoon ground nutmeg
¼ teaspoon kosher salt
¼ teaspoon freshly ground black pepper
1 cup Castelvetrano olives, pitted and sliced
⅓ cup grated Parmesan cheese

1. In a large stockpot of salted water, cook the pasta for about 8 to 10 minutes. Drain the pasta and reserve ¼ cup of the cooking liquid.
2. Meanwhile, heat the olive oil in a large skillet over medium heat. Add the garlic and red pepper and cook for 30 seconds, stirring constantly.
3. Add the parsley and cook for 1 minute, stirring constantly. Add the spinach, nutmeg, salt, and

pepper, and cook for 3 minutes, stirring occasionally, or until the spinach is wilted.
4. Add the cooked pasta and the reserved ¼ cup cooking liquid to the skillet. Stir in the olives and cook for about 2 minutes, or until most of the pasta water has been absorbed.
5. Remove from the heat and stir in the cheese before serving.

Per Serving

calories: 262 | fat: 4.0g | protein: 15.0g | carbs: 51.0g | fiber: 13.0g | sodium: 1180mg

Caprese Pasta with Roasted Asparagus

Prep time: 5 minutes | Cook time: 25 minutes | Serves 6

8 ounces (227 g) uncooked small pasta, like orecchiette (little ears) or farfalle (bow ties)

1½ pounds (680 g) fresh asparagus, ends trimmed and stalks chopped into 1-inch pieces

1½ cups grape tomatoes, halved

2 tablespoons extra-virgin olive oil

¼ teaspoon kosher salt

¼ teaspoon freshly ground black pepper

2 cups fresh Mozzarella, drained and cut into bite-size pieces (about 8 ounces / 227 g)

⅓ cup torn fresh basil leaves

2 tablespoons balsamic vinegar

1. Preheat the oven to 400°F (205°C).
2. In a large stockpot of salted water, cook the pasta for about 8 to 10 minutes. Drain and reserve about ¼ cup of the cooking liquid.
3. Meanwhile, in a large bowl, toss together the asparagus, tomatoes, oil, salt and pepper. Spread the mixture onto a large, rimmed

baking sheet and bake in the oven for 15 minutes, stirring twice during cooking.
4. Remove the vegetables from the oven and add the cooked pasta to the baking sheet. Mix with a few tablespoons of cooking liquid to help the sauce become smoother and the saucy vegetables stick to the pasta.
5. Gently mix in the Mozzarella and basil. Drizzle with the balsamic vinegar. Serve from the baking sheet or pour the pasta into a large bowl.

Per Serving

calories: 147 | fat: 3.0g | protein: 16.0g | carbs: 17.0g | fiber: 5.0g | sodium: 420mg

Garlic Shrimp Fettuccine

Prep time: 10 minutes | Cook time: 15 minutes | Serves 4 to 6

8 ounces (227 g) fettuccine pasta

¼ cup extra-virgin olive oil

3 tablespoons garlic, minced

1 pound (454 g) large shrimp, peeled and deveined

⅓ cup lemon juice

1 tablespoon lemon zest

½ teaspoon salt

½ teaspoon freshly ground black pepper

1. Bring a large pot of salted water to a boil. Add the fettuccine and cook for 8 minutes. Reserve ½ cup of the cooking liquid and drain the pasta.
2. In a large saucepan over medium heat, heat the olive oil. Add the garlic and sauté for 1 minute.
3. Add the shrimp to the saucepan and cook each side for 3 minutes. Remove the shrimp from the pan and set aside.
4. Add the remaining ingredients to the saucepan. Stir in the cooking liquid. Add the pasta and toss together to evenly coat the pasta.
5. Transfer the pasta to a serving dish and serve topped with the cooked shrimp.

Per Serving

calories: 615 | fat: 17.0g | protein: 33.0g | carbs: 89.0g | fiber: 4.0g | sodium: 407mg

Pesto Pasta

Prep time: 10 minutes | Cook time: 8 minutes | Serves 4 to 6

1 pound (454 g) spaghetti	½ teaspoon freshly ground black pepper
4 cups fresh basil leaves, stems removed	½ cup toasted pine nuts
3 cloves garlic	¼ cup lemon juice
1 teaspoon salt	½ cup grated Parmesan cheese
	1 cup extra-virgin olive oil

1. Bring a large pot of salted water to a boil. Add the spaghetti to the pot and cook for 8 minutes.
2. In a food processor, place the remaining ingredients, except for the olive oil, and pulse.
3. While the processor is running, slowly drizzle the olive oil through the top opening. Process until all the olive oil has been added.
4. Reserve ½ cup of the cooking liquid. Drain the pasta and put it into a large bowl. Add the pesto and cooking liquid to the bowl of pasta and toss everything together.

5. Serve immediately.

Per Serving

calories: 1067 | fat: 72.0g | protein: 23.0g | carbs: 91..0g | fiber: 6.0g | sodium: 817mg

Poultry and Meats

Lamb Kofta (Spiced Meatballs)

Prep time: 15 minutes | Cook time: 30 minutes | Serves 2

¼ cup walnuts

1 garlic clove

½ small onion

1 roasted piquillo pepper

2 tablespoons fresh mint

2 tablespoons fresh parsley

¼ teaspoon cumin

¼ teaspoon allspice

¼ teaspoon salt

Pinch cayenne pepper

8 ounces (227 g) lean ground lamb

1. Preheat the oven to 350ºF (180ºC). Line a baking sheet with aluminum foil.
2. In a food processor, combine the walnuts, garlic, onion, roasted pepper, mint, parsley, cumin, allspice, salt, and cayenne pepper. Pulse about 10 times to combine everything.
3. Transfer the spice mixture to a large bowl and add the ground lamb. With your hands or a spatula, mix the spices into the lamb.

4. Roll the lamb into 1½-inch balls (about the size of golf balls).
5. Arrange the meatballs on the prepared baking sheet and bake for 30 minutes, or until cooked to an internal temperature of 165ºF (74ºC).
6. Serve warm.

Per Serving

calories: 409 | fat: 22.9g | protein: 22.0g | carbs: 7.1g | fiber: 3.0g | sodium: 428mg

Fish and Seafood

Baked Salmon with Tarragon Mustard Sauce

Prep time: 5 minutes | Cook time: 12 minutes | Serves 4

1¼ pounds (567 g) salmon fillet (skin on or removed), cut into 4 equal pieces

¼ cup Dijon mustard

¼ cup avocado oil mayonnaise

Zest and juice of ½ lemon

2 tablespoons chopped fresh tarragon

½ teaspoon salt

¼ teaspoon freshly ground black pepper

4 tablespoons extra-virgin olive oil, for serving

1. Preheat the oven to 425ºF (220ºC). Line a baking sheet with parchment paper.
2. Arrange the salmon pieces on the prepared baking sheet, skin-side down.
3. Stir together the mustard, avocado oil mayonnaise, lemon zest and juice, tarragon, salt, and pepper in a small bowl. Spoon the mustard mixture over the salmon.

4. Bake for 10 to 12 minutes, or until the top is golden and salmon is opaque in the center.
5. Divide the salmon among four plates and drizzle each top with 1 tablespoon of olive oil before serving.

Per Serving

calories: 386 | fat: 27.7g | protein: 29.3g | carbs: 3.8g | fiber: 1.0g | sodium: 632mg

Baked Lemon Salmon

Prep time: 5 minutes | Cook time: 20 minutes | Serves 4

¼ teaspoon dried thyme

½ teaspoon freshly ground black pepper

Zest and juice of ½ lemon

1 pound (454 g) salmon fillet

Nonstick cooking spray

¼ teaspoon salt

1. Preheat the oven to 425ºF (220ºC). Coat a baking sheet with nonstick cooking spray.
2. Mix together the thyme, lemon zest and juice, salt, and pepper in a small bowl and stir to incorporate.
3. Arrange the salmon, skin-side down, on the coated baking sheet. Spoon the thyme mixture over the salmon and spread it all over.
4. Bake in the preheated oven for about 15 to 20 minutes, or until the fish flakes apart easily. Serve warm.

Per Serving

calories: 162 | fat: 7.0g | protein: 23.1g | carbs: 1.0g | fiber: 0g | sodium: 166mg

Glazed Broiled Salmon

Prep time: 5 minutes | Cook time: 5 to 10 minutes | Serves 4

4 (4-ounce / 113-g) salmon fillets

3 tablespoons miso paste

2 tablespoons raw honey

1 teaspoon coconut aminos

1 teaspoon rice vinegar

1. Preheat the broiler to High. Line a baking dish with aluminum foil and add the salmon fillets.
2. Whisk together the miso paste, honey, coconut aminos, and vinegar in a small bowl. Pour the glaze over the fillets and spread it evenly with a brush.
3. Broil for about 5 minutes, or until the salmon is browned on top and opaque. Brush any remaining glaze over the salmon and broil for an additional 5 minutes if needed. The cooking time depends on the thickness of the salmon.
4. Let the salmon cool for 5 minutes before serving.

Per Serving

calories: 263 | fat: 8.9g | protein: 30.2g | carbs: 12.8g | fiber: 0.7g | sodium: 716mg

Baked Salmon with Basil and Tomato

Prep time: 10 minutes | Cook time: 20 minutes | Serves 2

2 (6-ounce / 170-g) boneless salmon fillets

1 tablespoon dried basil

1 tomato, thinly sliced

1 tablespoon olive oil

2 tablespoons grated Parmesan cheese

Nonstick cooking spray

1. Preheat the oven to 375°F (190°C). Line a baking sheet with a piece of aluminum foil and mist with nonstick cooking spray.
2. Arrange the salmon fillets onto the aluminum foil and scatter with basil. Place the tomato slices on top and drizzle with olive oil. Top with the grated Parmesan cheese.
3. Bake for about 20 minutes, or until the flesh is opaque and it flakes apart easily.
4. Remove from the oven and serve on a plate.

Per Serving

calories: 403 | fat: 26.5g | protein: 36.3g | carbs: 3.8g | fiber: 0.1g | sodium: 179mg

Honey-Mustard Roasted Salmon

Prep time: 5 minutes | Cook time: 15 to 20 minutes | Serves 4

2 tablespoons whole-grain mustard

2 garlic cloves, minced

1 tablespoon honey

¼ teaspoon salt

¼ teaspoon freshly ground black pepper

1 pound (454 g) salmon fillet

Nonstick cooking spray

1. Preheat the oven to 425ºF (220ºC). Coat a baking sheet with nonstick cooking spray.
2. Stir together the mustard, garlic, honey, salt, and pepper in a small bowl.
3. Arrange the salmon fillet, skin-side down, on the coated baking sheet. Spread the mustard mixture evenly over the salmon fillet.
4. Roast in the preheated oven for 15 to 20 minutes, or until it flakes apart easily and reaches an internal temperature of 145ºF (63ºC).
5. Serve hot.

Per Serving

calories: 185 | fat: 7.0g | protein: 23.2g | carbs: 5.8g | fiber: 0g | sodium: 311mg

Baked Fish with Pistachio Crust

Prep time: 10 minutes | Cook time: 15 to 20 minutes | Serves 4

½ cup extra-virgin olive oil, divided

1 pound (454 g) flaky white fish (such as cod, haddock, or halibut), skin removed

½ cup shelled finely chopped pistachios

½ cup ground flaxseed

Zest and juice of 1 lemon, divided

1 teaspoon ground cumin

1 teaspoon ground allspice

½ teaspoon salt

¼ teaspoon freshly ground black pepper

1. Preheat the oven to 400ºF (205ºC).
2. Line a baking sheet with parchment paper or aluminum foil and drizzle 2 tablespoons of olive oil over the sheet, spreading to evenly coat the bottom.
3. Cut the fish into 4 equal pieces and place on the prepared baking sheet.

4. In a small bowl, combine the pistachios, flaxseed, lemon zest, cumin, allspice, salt, and pepper. Drizzle in ¼ cup of olive oil and stir well.
5. Divide the nut mixture evenly on top of the fish pieces. Drizzle the lemon juice and remaining 2 tablespoons of olive oil over the fish and bake until cooked through, 15 to 20 minutes, depending on the thickness of the fish.
6. Cool for 5 minutes before serving.

Per Serving

calories: 509 | fat: 41.0g | protein: 26.0g | carbs: 9.0g | fiber: 6.0g | sodium: 331mg

Sole Piccata with Capers

Prep time: 10 minutes | Cook time: 17 minutes | Serves 4

1 teaspoon extra-virgin olive oil	2 tablespoons all-purpose flour
4 (5-ounce / 142-g) sole fillets, patted dry	2 cups low-sodium chicken broth
3 tablespoons almond butter	Juice and zest of ½ lemon
2 teaspoons minced garlic	2 tablespoons capers

1. Place a large skillet over medium-high heat and add the olive oil.
2. Sear the sole fillets until the fish flakes easily when tested with a fork, about 4 minutes on each side. Transfer the fish to a plate and set aside.
3. Return the skillet to the stove and add the butter.
4. Sauté the garlic until translucent, about 3 minutes.
5. Whisk in the flour to make a thick paste and cook, stirring constantly, until the mixture is golden brown, about 2 minutes.

6. Whisk in the chicken broth, lemon juice and zest.
7. Cook for about 4 minutes until the sauce is thickened.
8. Stir in the capers and serve the sauce over the fish.

Per Serving

calories: 271 | fat:13.0g | protein: 30.0g | carbs: 7.0g | fiber: 0g | sodium: 413mg

Haddock with Cucumber Sauce

Prep time: 10 minutes | Cook time: 10 minutes | Serves 4

¼ cup plain Greek yogurt
½ scallion, white and green parts, finely chopped
½ English cucumber, grated, liquid squeezed out
2 teaspoons chopped fresh mint
1 teaspoon honey
Sea salt and freshly ground black pepper, to taste
4 (5-ounce / 142-g) haddock fillets, patted dry
Nonstick cooking spray

1. In a small bowl, stir together the yogurt, cucumber, scallion, mint, honey, and a pinch of salt. Set aside.
2. Season the fillets lightly with salt and pepper.
3. Place a large skillet over medium-high heat and spray lightly with cooking spray.
4. Cook the haddock, turning once, until it is just cooked through, about 5 minutes per side.
5. Remove the fish from the heat and transfer to plates.
6. Serve topped with the cucumber sauce.

Per Serving

calories: 164 | fat: 2.0g | protein: 27.0g | carbs: 4.0g | fiber: 0g | sodium: 104mg

Crispy Herb Crusted Halibut

Prep time: 10 minutes | Cook time: 20 minutes | Serves 4

4 (5-ounce / 142-g) halibut fillets, patted dry
Extra-virgin olive oil, for brushing
½ cup coarsely ground unsalted pistachios
1 tablespoon chopped fresh parsley
1 teaspoon chopped fresh basil
1 teaspoon chopped fresh thyme
Pinch sea salt
Pinch freshly ground black pepper

1. Preheat the oven to 350ºF (180ºC). Line a baking sheet with parchment paper.
2. Place the fillets on the baking sheet and brush them generously with olive oil.
3. In a small bowl, stir together the pistachios, parsley, basil, thyme, salt, and pepper.
4. Spoon the nut mixture evenly on the fish, spreading it out so the tops of the fillets are covered.
5. Bake in the preheated oven until it flakes when pressed with a fork, about 20 minutes.
6. Serve immediately.

Per Serving

calories: 262 | fat: 11.0g | protein: 32.0g | carbs: 4.0g | fiber: 2.0g | sodium: 77mg

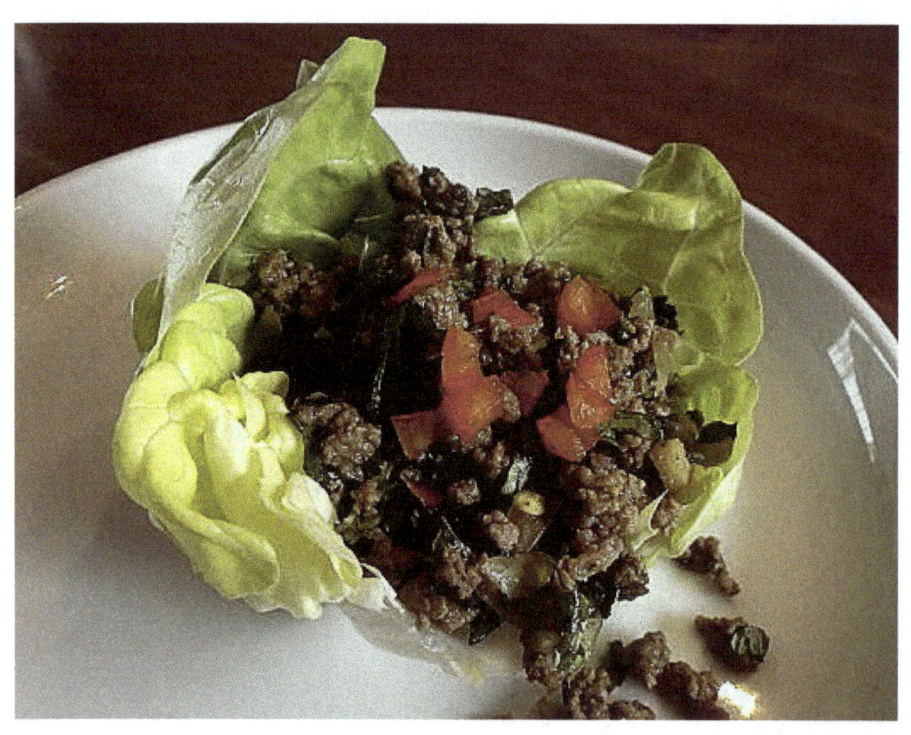

www.ingramcontent.com/pod-product-compliance
Lightning Source LLC
Chambersburg PA
CBHW070735030426
42336CB00013B/1977